Dedicated to a Great Friend, Colleague & Physician
Dr. Mark C. Johnson (1951-2024)
A Man of Rare Vision and Undying Inspiration

BARRY KRAKOW, MD

FAST ASLEEP

Advanced Guide
for Sleep Hygiene

The New Sleepy Times
NST

Cover: Bukovero, bukovero.com
Interior Formatting: Edge of Water Designs, edgeofwater.com
eBook designer: Laura Kincaid, Ten Thousand | Editing + Book Design,
www.tenthousand.co.uk

ISBNs: 978-0-9715869-4-9 (Paperback)
         978-0-9715869-5-6 (eBook)

LCCN: 2024923188

TABLE OF CONTENTS

PREFACE

In the original version of this book in 2002, I wanted my readers to know how I personally experienced the misery and frustration of insomnia. My first episodes with insomnia were minor – I could not fall asleep before the first day of school for most of my childhood. That was it. But in my twenties and thirties, I noticed occasional difficulties falling asleep at night. This subsided in medical school and residency as I was so painfully sleep deprived, I could sleep anywhere and everywhere, including cadaver tables (empty ones, of course.)

In my late thirties and early forties, it returned in mild form, and I simply made good use of my unslept hours by writing…research papers and ultimately books about insomnia and nightmares. In my mid-forties I developed moderate and occasionally severe insomnia, ironically enough only a few years after completing my formal training and board certification in sleep disorders medicine.

For the next five years, I tried everything short of sedatives to fix the problem, and in 1998 I discovered several cures for my insomnia of which a key component comprised what I now term advanced sleep hygiene.

Nearly a decade earlier, I had been instructing crime victims and other trauma survivors plagued with some of the worst insomnia problems imaginable on how to apply the principles and practice of advanced sleep hygiene. Many of these individuals suffered from other problems affecting their sleep, both mental and physical sleep conditions, and by addressing these aspects, they reached more comprehensive cures. During these years, I traveled a similar path and looking back now, I see my progress directly hinged on first mastering and applying an advanced sleep hygiene strategy.

Most people, although certainly not all, need to crawl before they walk, and perhaps we all need to walk before we run. Just so, advanced sleep hygiene can help virtually every type of insomniac improve sleeplessness, and most importantly, move closer toward a full recovery of normal sleep. For some people with mild or moderate insomnia, advanced sleep hygiene may be a cure-all.

For whatever reason and to whatever extent you suffer from insomnia, there is a distinct possibility a cure for your problem is attainable. And, in my personal and professional experience, as a first step towards this cure, I encourage you to closely examine and apply the principles of advanced sleep hygiene.

In this new version of the original book, you will find more instructions and updates that I believe will offer smoother sailing through the turbulent waters of sleeplessness.

Barry Krakow, MD
Savannah, GA 2024

INTRODUCTION

To understand why you may not fall asleep or stay asleep is a fairly easy knot to untangle. The more difficult part is learning how and when to apply specific remedies to reduce or eliminate your insomnia. For example, suppose you discover your sleeplessness is aggravated by clock-watching when you monitor how much sleep you are missing while lying awake in bed. Clock-watching is a common behavior among insomniacs, whether the sleep loss is caused by nightmares, depression, shift work, arthritic pains, other mental and physical disorders, or just about any other thing you might imagine. For most insomniacs who pay too much attention to the clock, there's a 95% chance it's fueling or worsening their sleeplessness.

Now, if I were to ask you to switch your clock so it faced the wall or to move the timepiece out of the bedroom entirely, it often turns out to be easier said than done. In other words, this BEHAVIOR (clock-watching) is simple to define, and it's been scientifically linked to insomnia. Yet, if I suggested a NEW BEHAVIOR (turn the clock face to the wall), would you readily accept this proposal? In my clinical experience, when you've agonized over sleepless nights for a long time, this simple instruction doesn't resonate. It takes time (pun intended) to appreciate how your attitude toward time monitoring plays a critically important role in recovering your normal sleep.

In my professional experience, this behavioral recommendation (avoid clock-watching) would be akin to telling overweight individuals all they really need to do is stop eating so much food. We know when you eat less, you'll lose weight, but so what! The real dilemma is learning the why and the how of not eating so much, and for many people it takes—you guessed it—time to figure out.

If the dilemma you face were analogous to crossing a river, which now seems overwhelming, your energy and motivation emerge when you find instructions to build a boat or a bridge.

Advanced sleep hygiene is the self-help tactical plan to construct this bridge. In other words, this book goes beyond a simplistic behavioral approach. That is, while I offer up standard, practical and essential sleep hygiene solutions, I also want to teach you a new way of thinking about the problem of insomnia. And, I sincerely believe this new way of thinking, including innovative sleep solutions, will lead you to apply this knowledge with greater confidence in treating your own sleeplessness.

As you learn to recognize all your sleep-negating BEHAVIORS, at the same time I will unmask for you a much more potent set of influences that play havoc with your sleep. These cognitive elements include: Thoughts, Ideas, Attitudes and Beliefs; and ultimately these mental processes help or hinder your quest to overcome insomnia. In fact, with respect to the BEHAVIOR (stop clock watching), it is the combination of COGNITIVE and BEHAVIORAL strategies that most effectively fixes your sleeplessness.

Advanced sleep hygiene takes into account all these factors to personally tailor the program to fit your specific set of sleep issues.

To reiterate, many patients with insomnia struggle to not

look at the clock, even *after* they've turned it to face the wall. Thus, what looks like a quick fix, isn't at all. But, when we add a COGNITIVE strategy to this NEW BEHAVIOR, the Sandman will soon be whispering in your ear.

———

As a bonus to your efforts, please take advantage of our Substack newsletter www.fastasleep.substack.com. Looking forward to a new podcast as well as a live Q & A series, where as always, we emphasize the mind-body approach to sleep disorders. Hope you'll visit us soon.

1

Is Your Bedroom the Enemy?

QUICK GUIDE

Problem: You arrive in the bedroom sleepy only to feel wide awake as soon as your head hits the pillow.

Cause: You've developed the habit of connecting your bedroom with mental alertness, which thwarts your natural ability to fall asleep.

Solution: Leave the bedroom and return once you feel sleepy again.

You're tired, exhausted, ready to drop. It's three yawns past 11 o'clock and blessed sleep is just around the corner in your bedroom. You plop into bed, pull up the covers, roll over once, twice, settle down and then...

...unbelievably, you're wide awake!

This is one of the most classic forms of insomnia. At the

moment of truth, it seems like you're about to fall asleep. Even before you land on the mattress, you can imagine nothing else but your head hitting the pillow followed by a visit from the Sandman.

Instead, you awaken, and more often than not, you spend another twenty, thirty and sometimes more than sixty minutes trying to get to sleep. Worse, you worry about how awful the next day might be. No matter how much you hoped to accomplish, despite all your best plans, you expect you'll be dragging around much of the day warding off fatigue, exhaustion and sometimes a genuine desire to fall asleep.

To add insult to injury, you ask yourself "why does this happen to me? Why can't I do what so many others seem to be able to do quite naturally—fall asleep and stay asleep?" There's almost a sense of guilt or blame for not getting the job done. It's as if sleep has become something you must perform. In a real sense, anxiety performance occurs regularly at bedtime, adding to your self-consciousness and aggravation about the sleeplessness, and in turn, making things worse.

So, the above scenario exemplifies how these thoughts undermine your sleep and aggravate your insomnia. The good news about this type of insomnia is it will almost always respond, in part, to the principles and practice of sleep hygiene.

Basic sleep hygiene encompasses many of the behaviors and habits in your daily life that affect your ability to sleep.

Overall, good sleep hygiene means creating an environment for yourself that promotes sound sleep. This environment includes physical things, like the type of mattress you sleep on or the degree of light in your bedroom. It includes mental things such as learning to trust yourself to fall asleep. Most of all, proper sleep hygiene means learning how to establish a VERY STRONG AND POSITIVE ASSOCIATION OR CONNECTION BETWEEN YOUR BEDROOM AND GOOD SLEEP.

If you've experienced the aggravation of becoming alert once you've entered your bedroom, then your **connection** between the bed and sleep is no longer optimal. Instead, somewhere in your mind and body, you develop nervousness about your ability to sleep well. Therefore, when you enter the bedroom, thoughts and feelings are triggered that wake you up instead of letting you doze off.

By using this newer, more advanced sleep hygiene program, you will learn how to trust your ability to fall asleep and stay asleep by **re-creating a positive connection between the bedroom and sleep**.

Step 1: Ask yourself how you feel about getting up out of bed and leaving the bedroom whenever you have difficulty falling asleep or staying asleep? Your answer to this question sheds light on your personal view of your sleep problem, so it may be worth pondering for a moment.

We shall explore many more questions and find useful answers throughout the book.

2

SLEEPY OR TIRED?
KNOW THE DIFFERENCE

QUICK GUIDE

Problem: Your ability to distinguish between genuine sleepiness and the feeling of fatigue or tiredness is blurred, creating confusion about when to go to sleep.

Cause: You no longer experience the natural sequence of feeling first tired, then sleepy before dozing off.

Solution: Ask yourself during the day: "am I sleepy?" or "am I tired?" until you appreciate the distinction, then monitor these feelings near your bedtime.

Do you know the difference between feeling sleepy and feeling tired? This distinction may seem obvious; however, it is a critical one for someone who suffers from insomnia.

Have you ever found yourself sitting quietly after lunch and noticed a strong feeling you might doze off?

That's true sleepiness. When you feel sleepy, there is a definite sense of drowsiness, often quite pleasurable. Your body slumps into a state of relaxation, and your mind drifts away from wakefulness into a hazier consciousness. If you try to stay awake or try to work while sleepy, a constant struggle ensues between the sleepiness, signaling the pleasure to be gained from nodding off versus your attempt to remain alert. A battle line is drawn, across which two opposing forces tug at you. And, at the end of the day if sleepiness wins out, the genuine pleasure of falling asleep proves to be one of life's most consistently satisfying experiences.

Fatigue or tiredness is very different than sleepiness; your body and mind feel worn out or overused. When fatigued but needing to work, a constant sense of discomfort nags at the back of your mind or permeates through the muscles of your body. There is no pleasure involved in feeling tired unless you stop what you're doing and allow yourself rest. Even then, rest may be unrewarding if you believe you really need to sleep, yet slumber will not come or is not permitted in these circumstances.

In the overwhelming majority of instances, it is essential to expect sleepiness to precede and facilitate sleep; whereas, fatigue or tiredness may yield a very inconsistent relationship with your ability to fall asleep.

As we move down the path toward healthy sleep, all the things we talk about are geared toward helping you appreciate and regain your natural ability to **feel sleepy**. Once you trust this feeling of sleepiness, healthy sleep patterns will be reestablished more rapidly.

As another step in this direction, take a moment right now and ask yourself these questions:

Do I feel sleepy?

Do I feel tired?

Do I feel alert?

You probably recognize instances in which you feel each of these three conditions separately, and in various combinations, and that's normal. For now, it could prove valuable to permit yourself the opportunity to tease out these feelings and sensations in more specific ways. Near bedtime, for example, when you appreciate you feel more sleepy than alert, there's an excellent chance you can *let* yourself fall asleep. On the other hand, as bedtime approaches if you notice feeling more tired than sleepy, it may prove difficult to try to sleep; in fact, it may be counterproductive to even attempt sleep.

If you feel tired, particularly when your fatigue has been generated by an active lifestyle of work and/or play, then sleepiness should follow. That a sleepy feeling does not follow on the footsteps of fatigue is at the heart of most insomnia problems. For some reason, this natural next step in the sequence from fatigue to sleepiness does not occur. Your mind or your body (usually both) learned to fight this progression; instead, you maintain a feeling of tiredness that no longer permits the pleasure of drowsiness to herald the need and desire for sleep.

When you learn to let tiredness take its natural course to sleepiness, your effort is almost 99% complete—sleep is not far off.

Unless you have suffered from lifelong, night after night insomnia (which is rare by the way), at some point you must have engaged in normal and successful sleep habits. As such, it is likely at least a few times in your life you felt sleepiness as a natural thing prior to sleep. Nodding off was easy and a genuine pleasure. During these times, this natural ability promoted a very strong and healthy connection between sleep and your bedroom.

With insomnia, from whatever the cause, this once healthy association becomes weaker and inconsistent. Therefore, I would ask you again to imagine how it might feel to get up out of bed and leave the bedroom when you notice you are feeling tired but not sleepy. This step can be attempted regardless of whether the difficulty occurs at bedtime or in the middle of the night.

Conversely, if you *only* feel tired while attempting to doze off, you continue to weaken your connection to the bedroom as a place for slumber. When you consider this sleep hygiene approach, recognize that by leaving the bedroom on the occasion of sleeplessness, you take the cause of your insomnia *out* of the bedroom. When you return, *leave it* outside where it can no longer interfere with your sleep.

3

MAKE YOUR BEDROOM
SLEEPER-FRIENDLY

QUICK GUIDE

Problem: You can fall asleep in other rooms, even other homes or hotels, but not in your own bed or bedroom.

Cause: You learned several negative associations between your *own* bed and other waking behaviors that literally teach you to remain awake in your *own* bedroom.

Solution: Use your bedroom only for sleep and nothing else until you consistently feel sleepy prior to bedtime.

———

If you ate pizza late in the evening and then had a nightmare after going to bed, would you wonder if this snack triggered your disturbing dream? Some people speculate about these types of connections, but what if the next week, you ate pizza again and had another bad dream. Your tendency to wonder whether the two things were connected would likely increase.

Now suppose you ate pizza a third time over this short time span; it would be easy to imagine you might have more than a passing thought about what you might dream. If you had another nightmare is the pizza to blame?

The answer is a definite yes and no.

No scientific evidence proves pizza has any impact whatsoever on your dreams (thank goodness!). However, once your mind draws an association between pizza and bad dreams, just a single bite stimulates thoughts and feelings in your waking consciousness that could trigger unpleasant dreams while asleep. The pizza serves as a catalyst, not because of anything in the ingredients, but simply the image or taste of pizza draws your memory back to the previous experiences with nightmares.

A connection was formed between pizza and nightmares. Likewise, the connections you develop between your ability to fall asleep and your sleep environment ultimately determine your success in achieving healthy sleep.

At a younger age, most associations developed naturally. You didn't spend much time, if any, thinking about what to do to get to sleep. In most instances, you felt tired, then sleepy, and then you went to sleep.

Over the course of your life, usually during times of stress, you learned new associations that conflict with these natural tendencies toward good sleep. These new associations generate negative attitudes, some more conscious than others, weakening your confidence in your sleep habits.

The primary negative association, conscious or otherwise, is the belief your bed and bedroom are no longer an obvious place to go to sleep and stay asleep. This association can be so strong that even if you were feeling very sleepy in the living room, you automatically come to full alertness when you walk into your bedroom. As a result, sooner or later, you find yourself falling asleep in different places in your house, like the living room sofa or in the family room watching TV.

In time, you feel tremendously frustrated when you are sleepy in one part of your home, only to discover this pleasurable feeling is replaced in your bedroom in the blink of an eye with a sudden surge of alertness. More than frustrating, it is sometimes maddening, especially if you've spent a very active day at work or at play and believe you've earned a good night of slumber.

You most certainly do deserve a good night of sleep, many in fact, so hang in there and consider the following:

If you find yourself able to fall asleep in another room of the house, yet struggle doing so in your bedroom, it is almost certain you've developed a primary problem initiating sleep due to negative associations. When I interview patients with insomnia, one of the first questions I ask is if they can recall recent travel or spending the night at someone else's home. Often, though not always, someone who complains of not being able to fall asleep in his or her own bed will report no difficulty in dozing off in a hotel or at a friend's house.

When we examine this person's insomnia in more depth with a polysomnogram—an all-night laboratory test to evaluate sleep—this type of insomnia, that is, a delay in falling asleep, may not occur because the new laboratory environment holds no negative associations for the insomniac. It is quite common, and perhaps embarrassingly so, for the patient to awaken from the lab and admit she never slept so well in recent memory.

So, if you can fall asleep in one place, but dread your own bed, how do you fix this problem? Better said, how do you break this cycle?

Do you remember as a child or some other time when you played with a little straw toy called the Chinese Finger Puzzle. You inserted a finger from each hand into the ends of the short straw tube, but as you probably remember the more you tugged at each end, the harder it became to remove your fingers. In fact, only when you relaxed your fingers and stopped trying so hard would you find release from the tube. In effect, you learned how to *let* your fingers escape.

With insomnia, it is crucial to stop trying so hard to fall asleep.

It will happen if you *let it*…and, you can improve your chances by bringing genuine sleepiness back to the bedroom where it belongs. On a good night when you feel sleepy in bed, obviously let yourself doze off. But on a bad night, when not sleepy in bed, consider getting up and leaving the bedroom temporarily.

At first, this get up and go technique proves confusing to many insomniacs, because they are uncertain about how long it should take to initially get sleepy and doze off. For starters, we say it's reasonable to use a window of 20 to 40 minutes (just estimate, don't watch the clock). Nevertheless, if you jump into bed and within 5 minutes you know you're not going to sleep anytime soon, then the very big question must arise, "why not get up now?" At this point, it should sound reasonable to get up and leave the bed and bedroom; and, in most circumstances, this step is the right move.

Generally, your goal is to wait for sleepiness to return, then go back to bed. By doing so, you re-build the positive connection between sleep and the bedroom that leads you to rediscover your natural ability to fall asleep.

Finally, let's mention something here about staying asleep. Many people fall asleep without much difficulty, but then routinely awaken in the middle of the night. They believe their **problem** is in staying asleep, but I would suggest the true problem remains that of falling asleep.

The reason returning to sleep may be the more helpful view of the problem is that *everyone* awakens from sleep throughout the night and with some regularity. Good sleepers, however, have little difficulty dozing off again to resume sleep whether or not they recall these brief awakenings that could easily number five or ten per night.

While various causes for awakenings may need to be investigated, early on it is more practical and useful to think of middle of the night insomnia as difficulty in falling asleep or if you prefer, falling back asleep. Virtually all the tips offered in this book apply to both falling asleep at bedtime and in the middle of the night.

4

Time Is Not of the Essence

QUICK GUIDE

Problem: Unwitting alerting behaviors are disrupting your ability to fall asleep or stay asleep.

Cause: Commonplace negative associations have developed such as looking at the clock to monitor how long it takes you to fall asleep or how much sleep you anticipate getting.

Solution: Turn the clock to face the wall, put your phone out of reach, or remove both from the bedroom.

Any negative associations between sleep and bedroom may seem challenging to deal with, yet in practicality they are easy to solve because the solution is as simple as:

USE YOUR BEDROOM ONLY FOR SLEEP . . .

. . . OR MAKING LOVE.

Perhaps you believe you are already doing so, but there are many subtle ways of defeating this singular principle. A prime example is clock-watching. If you are disturbed or frustrated by the length of time it takes to fall asleep, you may be the type of person who monitors exactly how much sleep you're losing. Or, if you awaken in the middle of the night, you developed the habit of turning over to see what time it is, so you can calculate how much possible sleep time remains...if you could get back to sleep.

In both instances, your brain is engaged in an alerting type of behavior. When else do you look at the clock? Perhaps to check the time to: Get to work? Get to school? Break for lunch? Make an appointment? Watch a favorite TV program? The list goes on. Checking the clock and thinking about time is a common waking behavior, occurring all day long and often right up until bedtime when you might check to see how late it is before retiring.

Checking your phone or looking at a clock, then, has a very strong association with activity and schedules and all sorts of daily life routines. Therefore, you could say it has everything to do with *not* falling asleep or staying asleep! Yet, given this knowledge, many insomniacs continue to monitor the clock and in so doing continue to fuel their insomnia.

Let's take a moment to look at the less obvious connections between time and clock-watching to figure out why insomniacs balk at turning the clock to face the wall.

Surely, we know you look at the clock to make decisions about what's going on with your sleep during the night. But, the far greater premise driving this behavior is an unshakeable belief *more* sleep must be the ultimate goal.

And how couldn't we be driven there after hearing (for the 500th time) "get 8 hours of sleep per night?" Anything fewer than

8 hours feels like you're coming up short.

Spoiler Alert: The *quantity* of your sleep can't hold a candle to the importance and benefit from the *quality* of your sleep (to be continued)!

Forecasting quantity keeps us overly concerned about the amount of sleep time we are supposed to get, which then demands we count the minutes in the middle of the night and calculate the number of hours we still might get. So, not only does time mess up our sleep by having us spend time counting and not sleeping, but time pervades our whole perspective about sleep and is a setup for failure.

Time issues reflect even deeper concerns and fears about our lives. On a profound note, the questions that lurk within each of us might be: Will I have enough time to accomplish all that I want to with my life? How much time do I really have to accomplish these things? On a pragmatic scale, there is the constant hurry-and-worry lifestyle infecting modern society; instead of the old saw, less is more, our new mantra is more is more. In truth, there is only so much "more" you can pack into any single day, and if you fail to meet your daily objectives, it is not uncommon to bring all that unsatisfied energy with you into the bedroom where you might mistakenly believe you can "finish your work."

Such an attitude completely negates the purpose of the bed and bedroom and of sleep itself. In this hectic and frazzled world, good sleep is not only necessary, but it is also a well-deserved break from our incredibly busy, hurry-and-worry lives. The bedroom therefore ought to be a sanctuary, a special place to shut out and turn off the misery and hassles of the world outside. It ought to be a place to tune in to the restorative and healing power of sleep.

Finally, clock watching is one of the best examples of how

you are *not* USING YOUR BEDROOM ONLY FOR SLEEP. While it might seem like a ludicrously simple treatment, I have helped hundreds of individuals completely overcome their sleeplessness by asking them to turn their clock to face the wall or to remove it altogether from the bedroom. Same for the phone. No other therapy was required, and the insomnia departed once they stopped checking the time.

If clock-watching is a regular activity in your nightly routine, it's likely you've been doing it for a long time. Regardless of how long you've engaged in time-checking, eliminating this alerting behavior from your bedroom will prove a major step forward in your recovery of good sleep.

Before proceeding, however, it is imperative to appreciate the connections you've developed between time and sleep. Once these associations are clearer, you will find it easier to turn the clock to the wall or to place the phone out of reach.

One last tip: if you can't see a clock or phone, you could still listen for noises outside like traffic or roosters, check the light coming thru the window or detect other clues about the current hour. This more subtle time monitoring causes the same problems as clock-watching and must be avoided.

Seriously, you have no time, any time, for TIME in your bedroom!

5

KILL YOUR TELEVISION AND BANISH THE SCREENS

QUICK GUIDE

Problem: Television or screen images helped you fall asleep but no longer make you feel drowsy.

Cause: Despite boring programs on the tube or phone, you are accustomed to lying in bed watching a screen instead of lying in bed sleeping.

Solution: Do not watch TV or any screen in bed.

In treating insomnia with the principles of sleep hygiene, there are innumerable possibilities for negative connections that need to be addressed; and, it is well worth your while to investigate them all as each one serves as a cue blocking your natural sleepiness. As we explore these major and minor situations, behaviors and so forth, please bear in mind virtually all considerations relate back to the singular problem of learning to use your bedroom for something other than sleeping.

A rather obvious obstacle to sound sleep emerging during the last seventy years is the initial technology of the television and subsequent derivations commonly referred to as "screen time." TV has its own intrinsic drawbacks because it produces a passive relationship between the viewer and the tube, whereas other forms of activity yield a clearer sense of engaging in something of genuine benefit, be it work or play oriented.

While this passive effect of television produces drowsiness in some people, by and large, TV is something you attempt to do as a waking behavior: you seek to watch your favorite program, or to see a sporting event with a group of friends or to catch up on the latest soap opera melodrama.

Therefore, when you watch TV in your bedroom, it is likely to disrupt your healthy sleep habits. At first, TV could help you feel drowsy, particularly because of the incredibly boring programs now gracing the airwaves; but, unfortunately, over time, TV manifests the same impact as the clock. You are watching instead of sleeping, and your brain learns the bed is no longer simply for slumber.

Once your mind establishes this connection, regardless of what you watch on TV, you invoked an association that prevents natural sleepiness. Again, it is this type of association more than any other that goes to the heart of the problem, that is, your unconscious continues to receive a mixed message: watch TV and sleep, just like watch the clock and sleep, but you cannot do both at the same time. The conflict hidden in these mixed signals festers in your mind without much awareness, yet it wreaks havoc on your sleep. You must actively learn to choose sleep instead of choosing TV or clock watching.

Of course, the same holds for all the other forms of screen time.

Television and other screens also play a more active role in disrupting your sleep if you watch newscasts or sexually stimulating or action programming. These shows grab your attention, and some of the more horrific stories disrupt your sleep in more direct fashion by producing disturbing dreams. Self-serving, selfish and brazenly dishonest TV and media producers continue to attempt to discredit the research that demonstrates quite clearly TV pictures or other screens implant images into your mind, but both common sense and the facts speak otherwise.

In my own research specialty of helping people with chronic nightmares, I learned those afflicted with frequent bad dreams limit the amount of screen time they watch. They do so for the obvious reason to prevent the influx of disturbing images that could trigger a new round of nightmares.

Last, screen time also plays havoc with your circadian rhythm—the body's natural biological clock—that gears you up in the morning for a full day of activity and winds you down in the evening to prepare for sleep. Screen time interferes with this biological rhythm by encouraging you to stay up later. While most adults develop first sensations of sleepiness somewhere close to 9:00 PM or earlier, TV induces people to remain awake for hours beyond this time frame. For normal sleepers, a routine cycle of insufficient sleep is generated, but for insomniacs it throws a larger wrench into their circadian rhythm by teaching them to remain awake past midnight and thereby exacerbate existing difficulties with falling asleep. Eventually, the combination of late-night TV or screen use and insomnia produces an entirely new circadian rhythm of going to sleep in the wee hours of the night, which can reduce the insomniacs already shortened sleep cycle.

Television's effects on sleep are marked and omnipresent in our society. Learning how to limit the use of TV or other screens and removing them from the bedroom are two of the healthiest steps you can take in promoting better sleep hygiene and sounder sleep.

As needed, when you want to watch something close to bedtime, commit to watching it outside the bedroom.

6

You've Made Your Bed, But Don't Suffer in It

QUICK GUIDE

Problem: You spend a long time in bed lying awake either when you try to fall asleep or in the middle of the night.

Cause: You developed the most problematic connection between your bed and mental alertness, programming yourself to stay awake and not sleep in the bedroom.

Solution: Never spend more than a set, estimated period in bed awake (for example, twenty or forty or sixty minutes); if you're not asleep when the estimated time is up, leave the bedroom and return when you feel sleepy.

Reading in bed fits into a special category because it can help or hinder your ability to fall asleep. Some people swear by their use of light reading material in bed just a few minutes before lights out. Others feel enough stimulation to find themselves reading two hours later!

Your decision about whether to read in bed or not must be weighed with your practical experience. If it works, even though it would appear to fly in the face of the general principles of sleep hygiene, perhaps it is helping you relax and take your mind off the day's events or future worries.

If it doesn't work and exacerbates your difficulties with falling asleep, then reading is stimulating and alerting you and thwarting your natural sleepiness. *Outside of the bedroom*, however, reading is probably one of the best activities you can do as you await the return of drowsiness.

While social media, television, clock watching, and reading at length represent the most common negative associations that could interfere with falling asleep and staying asleep, many other actions may need to be addressed as well. If you use your bedroom as an office for paying bills, can you imagine what a bad connection you've built as you literally let financial stress and worries into your bed? In contrast, journaling to unwind from daily encounters may let you relax.

Social media, however, is now a major factor among insomnia causes as you are quite literally sharing your space with the world. Your brain may descend into a certain mode, some would call it a trance, that deceives you into a false sense of relaxation, that is actually stimulating and addictive. In sum, all these actions and behaviors must be examined, whenever you find yourself in bed *not* sleeping or making love.

Of all the possible negative situations, though, the simplest *and* worst for your sleep is **lying awake in bed.**

A TV, phone, clock or a book are external, physical objects that occupy your attention, prohibiting your natural tendency toward sleep; nevertheless, the internal processes of your mind and body ultimately determine whether or not you can shut off the day's events so drowsiness will lead you to sleep. If you choose to remain in bed *and* think, you are establishing the strongest possible connection between your bed and mental activity and alertness. In other words, your bedroom becomes a place no longer associated with sleeping; instead, your bed itself becomes a place to continue the day in your mind's eye.

Just as you would not go to your workplace to sleep, why would you enter your sleep-space to work?

This negative mental connection between bedroom and thinking is perhaps the most difficult habit to overcome for any insomniac, particularly because someone who suffers from sleeplessness may stay in bed for any number of reasons, all of which appear quite reasonable.

It is a myth that it's better to rest even if you can't get to sleep. Still, many can't imagine getting up out of bed because all they really want to do is sleep. Those who lie in bed with racing thoughts often feel powerless to stop them. Then, there are those who lie awake apparently without any thoughts whatsoever, but remain frozen to the mattress.

In response to this wide assortment of reasons for remaining awake in bed, sleep hygiene offers one simple challenge: GET UP OUT OF BED AND LEAVE THE BEDROOM UNTIL YOU FEEL SLEEPY!

This is the cornerstone of advanced sleep hygiene. And, while this specific advice seems to be a difficult pill to swallow, especially during the first few trials, it has proven time and again to be the single most effective component of any sleep promoting regimen for someone suffering from insomnia.

The advice to get up out of bed and leave the bedroom may sound drastic, but the connection your mind has made between sleep and wakefulness is exceedingly powerful. In no uncertain terms, to lie awake in bed, whether you think, don't think, rest or don't rest, your mind and body now believe the bed and the bedroom are places in which it's perfectly normal to remain awake . . . and suffer the distress of insomnia!

When you leave the bedroom and engage in some activity in another room reading, writing, eating a small snack, or even watching TV you are letting your mind know wakefulness occurs outside the bedroom, *not* in the bed. This new and healthier habit can be learned in a matter of days, sometimes a mere three days.

To repeat, the key is letting your natural sleepiness reassert itself so you return to the bedroom only when you feel drowsy. Then, if you were to lie down, but the sensation of wakefulness returned, you would be faced with the same challenge as before, that is, would you be willing to leave the bedroom yet again?

To some, this proves very frustrating, especially because this process may need repeating several times in the first few nights. These initial attempts, as challenging as they may appear, will often produce rapid success in learning to overcome the unhealthy habit of lying awake in bed.

In practice, suppose you had to get up out of bed and leave the bedroom not just once or twice, but three times? Can you imagine how taxing it would be to your sense of well-being? No doubt, it would feel like you were adding to your efforts to sleep. Fortunately, there is nothing harmful about this routine.

To the point, it is essential to realize: 1) lying in bed awake is harmful when your goal is to fall asleep; and 2) lying in bed awake for a lengthy time is rarely restful.

Imagine you had the choice of lying in bed for only six and one-half hours with a guarantee you would always sleep six hours, or you could lie in bed for ten hours with no guarantee of how many hours you might sleep. Which routine would you choose?

Your answer will tell you a lot about your own understanding of sleep and rest.

7

Quality, Not Quantity

QUICK GUIDE

Problem: Your sleep is light, superficial and unrestful.

Cause: Your total time in bed involves too much time awake, which then filters into your unconscious to fragment your actual sleep.

Solution: Focus on sleep quality, not quantity. Less time in bed will retrain your mind to facilitate deeper sleep.

———

If it surprises you a person who spends *less* time in bed gains better quality sleep, then please consider this example: two people both receive exactly six hours of sleep each night, but one lies in bed ten hours while the other spends only six and one-half hours there.

Will the six hours of actual sleep be the same for each person?

Most likely not. Why would the six hours prove different in each case? Let's explore the answer in some detail to reinforce the importance of not remaining in bed while awake.

Sleep, as we understand it with the relatively primitive technological tools we have at our disposal, appears to progress through a variety of stages during the course of a normal night's sleep. In non-medical terms, it is easiest to describe three types: deep sleep, light sleep and dream awareness sleep.

When a person is studied in a sleep lab with the polysomnogram, she is hooked up to numerous wires, probes and monitors to measure brain waves, eye movements, breathing, snoring, chin tension, heart rate, and chest, abdominal and leg movements. By monitoring all this information, we can establish how much time she spends in various sleep stages.

For most insomniacs, an inordinate amount of time is usually spent in lighter stages of sleep at the expense of both deep and dream awareness sleep. As you might imagine, the lack of adequate deep and dream stages partially explains why an insomniac often complains of feeling unrested. This complaint is legitimate and can easily be reproduced by anyone who attempts to sleep an entire night with loud and irritating music or other noises close to the bedside.

In other words, if you sleep *lightly* much of the time which unfortunately is standard for many insomniacs, then the actual number of total hours slept may be meaningless to you.

From medical-scientific research investigations, it can be clearly stated that:

The longer you remain in bed in a vain attempt to sleep, the more you disrupt your overall sleep and thereby limit deep and dream sleep.

The reason for this paradox is too much time in bed trying

to sleep yields the opposite, that is, too much time awake. Over the course of a night, a person who remains convinced of the need to spend more time in bed actually develops a problem called *sleep fragmentation.* In sleep medicine research, we know this fragmentation indicates you are alternating between stages of sleep and stages where the brain suffers arousals or full awakenings. To be clear, you may not be aware of these arousals that last less than a minute. Nonetheless, this alternating pattern literally blocks you from entering deeper sleep stages.

For example, even if you slept six hours while lying in bed for ten, you will have also experienced four hours of wakefulness. For reasons that are not completely understood, it appears this increase in time awake (the four hours) filters into your unconscious during your time asleep (the six hours). By repeating this process nightly, your mind distinguishes less and less between **being asleep and being awake**. The result is your sleep cycle spends more time in the lighter stages. At some point, your sleep becomes so superficial, you may think you're not even sleeping at all or perhaps for just a short period.

Sadly, this well-intentioned attempt to gain sufficient hours of slumber yields lighter sleep; and, as you futilely spend more time in bed, the vicious cycle continues or worsens.

The old saying, "less is more," speaks volumes to anyone suffering from insomnia, particularly those who have been troubled chronically by sleeplessness.

Sleep quality is the crucial factor in rehabilitating the insomniac. Learn to focus on the quality of sleep; even slight increases in your deep or dream sleep will usher in an entirely new and more satisfying perspective regarding your ability to obtain restful and refreshing slumber.

If you currently spend more than one or two hours in bed awake, then consider cutting down this time awake. Specifically, if you know you've been awake for about 75 minutes, then commit to only staying in bed for 60 minutes of awake time. Make this change during the next seven nights. Then, the second week cut it another 15 minutes per night, so now you're spending no more than 45 minutes awake in bed.

Goals may vary, but many insomniacs notice much deeper sleep once they can limit their awake time in bed to 30 minutes or less. Now, some can cut down their time in bed more rapidly, which is fine if you are eager to attempt such a drastic approach. It has been known to work miracles. For others who want to change at a slower pace, I recommend the more gradual approach, though surprisingly very small reductions to the time in bed sometimes markedly increases time asleep. In sum, decreased time in bed will generate sounder sleep, particularly as your time awake in bed decreases.

Remember, in this instance *less* really is *more*.

8

Losing Sleep Over Losing Sleep

QUICK GUIDE

Problem: You cannot go to sleep because you worry about not going to sleep. You are afraid you might be harming your health if you don't gain sufficient slumber.

Cause: Fear has many disguises: insomnia and fears about sleeplessness are very common.

Solution: No one has ever directly died from a loss of sleep; whereas losing sleep over losing sleep (LSOLS) guarantees you will lose more sleep. Instead, reflect on and seek to resolve other fears: work stress, relationship conflicts, health concerns. Usually, these difficulties are greater sources of fear that sabotage your sleep and lead to insomnia.

Does a shorter time in bed mean the insomniac is doomed to a life of shorter sleep? By all means no!

Still, practicing a shorter sleep cycle may be worthwhile during specific episodes of insomnia, and it may teach you how to not worry about your total sleep time. Moreover, by appreciating the importance of sleep quality, you may shift your focus away from your worries about hours of sleep.

The worries people develop about their sleep habits are genuine and often very emotional. The two most common feelings are the fear you will not be able to fall asleep and the fear you will be harmed by not obtaining enough sleep.

Let's examine both fears.

It is helpful to learn no one ever died directly from sleep loss. There is an extremely rare hereditary disorder known as Fatal Familial Insomnia, but this disease relates to severe brain degeneration, which causes the sleeplessness, not the reverse.

To be sure, people suffering chronic insomnia are more vulnerable to infections like colds or the flu. They may be prone to accidents, errors and mistakes, such as motor vehicle accidents or lapses in concentration or memory. However, any specific night of lost or diminished sleep is not likely to be directly harmful in a way that causes life-threatening health problems like heart attacks or strokes.

Despite hearing the above explanation, more severe insomniacs may latch onto an irrational fear of sleeplessness. The obsession grows so large, the insomniac "loses sleep over losing sleep (LSOLS)." This mindset must be directly targeted to re-order the person's thinking. For some, intensive psychotherapy or other interventions are needed to overcome the fixation.

In other forms of LSOLS, two points need to be reiterated and, in some cases closely scrutinized.

First, insomnia itself cannot directly cause injury. People in all walks of life combat occasional episodes of sleeplessness during situations with work, school, children crying at night, or other events. Some face regularly occurring sleep deprivation episodes similar to insomniacs. These folks respond to lost sleep by going about the next day's business, perhaps with greater fatigue, or with caffeinated drinks, or by napping. Further, no scientific reports show a single lost night of sleep results in deadly harm. After a lost night, it certainly would be prudent to avoid driving a car on a long-distance solo excursion, or to avoid other potentially dangerous settings.

Second, when an irrational fear about sleep arises, another fear almost always lurks beneath the surface, and this deeper fear only makes itself known as the insomnia, because sleeplessness is less threatening to the human mind. In my experience, deep-seated emotions typically disturbing ones, such as depression, anxiety, guilt, or anger are the underlying culprits fueling the fear. Without proper self-reflection to effectively cope with these stronger emotions, the individual is left to confront the problem of insomnia instead.

Depression can be a brutal and agonizing experience, inflicting more pain and misery than almost the worst imaginable physical pain. With physical pain there may appear to be a chance for relief at some point. With serious depression, often the individual feels hopeless—the future appears bleak without any promise of recovery. For these reasons, a person might grow to fear depression, especially if she has experienced it once and dreads the day she might be depressed again.

In such instances, the depressed person may develop an irrational fear of insomnia because of this deeper emotional distress and may need counseling to help connect and deal with the real fear.

The fear of not being able to fall asleep itself may fit into the category of LSOLS. Insomniacs who reach a state of exasperation often describe an intense frustration arising in the bedroom when attempting to doze. Again, this fear may be the sign of emotional turmoil. A classic case would be the individual who has been noticing stress at work. Anticipation of renewed conflict on a particular day may spark a genuine fear about returning to work; this fear is then displaced into a fear about not being able to go to sleep.

Some emotionally charged situations can be discussed with an attentive and compassionate person, such as a health care professional or a minister. Often, your primary doctor or sympathetic clergy would be the place to start. Short term counseling from a mental health therapist could also produce dramatic improvement in your ability to cope with the underlying conflict.

With respect to advanced sleep hygiene, it's important to realize irrational fears about insomnia are likely to thwart your straightforward efforts to reprogram your sleep patterns. On the other hand, recognize how the simple solutions offered through a sleep hygiene program may breathe enough confidence into your attitude to assist you in overcoming these troublesome fears.

To be sure, if you feel a real fear for safety in your sleep environment, then it is necessary to find a way to improve the conditions as best you can. No one should tell you to downplay such a fear, for when you are asleep you may be extremely vulnerable if someone or something poses a threat. In this instance, it is essential to take measures to enhance your safety. Steps might include better locks on doors and windows, installing a security alarm, owning a guard dog, or talking with good friends and neighbors who know your concerns and will check up on you. In some situations, while it may sound extreme (you must be the judge), a weapon of some sort could be what ultimately makes you feel secure in your bedroom.

In sum, if you have experienced too many bad nights to count, you may develop a fear about any single bad night's sleep. That is, you now believe regaining your healthy sleep is an all-or-nothing affair. Unless you sleep well every night, one bad night triggers weeks or months of insomnia. Not only is this view unrealistic, but also counterproductive. Everyone, good sleepers included, has some bad nights. Unfortunately, your memory of too many bad nights may cloud your perceptions, yielding unachievable desires for the perfect sleep. So, as your insomnia improves, please keep in mind a bad night of sleep does not invariably produce a domino effect.

Let me close with a caution: if you firmly believe your real-time fear is unequivocally about losing sleep, I encourage you to obtain either of my two books for a more detailed treatment analysis. Most recently, *Life Saving Sleep* (2023) and *Sound Sleep, Sound Mind* (2008) walk you through the deeper emotional factors that must be addressed to overcome LSOLS.

9

DOES YOUR SCHEDULE NEED
A WAKE-UP CALL?

QUICK GUIDE

Problem: Difficulty falling asleep creates havoc with your schedule if you fall out well beyond bedtime. A drive to sleep in until later the next morning may prove irresistible.

Cause: Your natural biological clock—the circadian rhythm—pushes you into a new, often undesirable routine.

Solution: Pick a set wakeup time and follow it seven days per week (allow no more than a one-hour difference on the weekends) even when you stay up late.

Let's return to bedtime and wakeup schedules, Benjamin Franklin's key to sleep hygiene. We've mentioned circadian rhythms, the body's biological timekeeper. Once you understand the general nature of this rhythm, you can apply this information to promote better sleep. In acknowledging the value of your innate biological clock, you will again notice the emphasis on sleep quality over total sleep time.

The circadian rhythm naturally establishes a pattern of being awake during the day and being asleep during the night, largely through changes in body temperature.

Your body's thermostat rises and remains higher during the day. At night, your temperature falls and remains low until near morning wake-up. Both the difference in temperature, higher vs. lower, and the changing nature of the temperature, rising and falling, are linked to your ability to be awake and stay awake as well as to your ability to fall asleep and stay asleep, respectively.

When you establish a consistent day-night rhythm, it yields a similar consistency in temperature patterns, which then facilitate alertness and sleepiness at proper times. The easiest way to help your body maintain a consistent rhythm is by setting a regular bedtime and wakeup time.

To be sure, you would welcome a regular sleep schedule, but sleeplessness thwarts your efforts. So, most insomniacs relate to the night owl syndrome, delaying bedtime later and later into the night for fear of another failed attempt at nodding off. And, if sleep does not commence until early morning, many doze well past normal wakeup times. This delay in falling asleep and in waking up trains your body to go to bed progressively later and allow for a progressively later wake up, too.

This cycle of delay becomes so chronic, poor sleepers perceive themselves as night people who only fall asleep in the middle of the night or even the early morning hours. In fact, they are partially correct because their circadian rhythms develop and sustain this night owl pattern.

Changing such a rhythm takes time and can be exceedingly frustrating. What's even more difficult to change is a chaotic rhythm jumping all around the clock, making the insomniac's lifestyle helter-skelter. In either of these situations where the body's rhythm has deviated far from the norm, it is usually more helpful for the patient to seek help from a sleep disorders specialist. A physician or psychologist who specializes in sleep medicine will have training and clinical experience in aiding the individual's recovery of a normal rhythm.

Most insomniacs do not reach this severe level of circadian disturbance; however, periodically they will notice enough variation in a sleep cycle to cause sporadic bed and wakeup times, which may be further compounded by erratic napping. Other examples of this problem would be staying up late or sleeping late on weekends, which will then influence the weekday schedule along a similar track.

Among insomniacs who complain about falling asleep at bedtime as their primary problem, trying to establish a regular routine is a nonstarter. Instead, the sensible strategy is to work backwards by committing to a regular wakeup time. If you establish this morning time *seven days per week*, it will produce enough regularity to influence if not entrain your bedtime as well.

Let's use the example of a 7:00 AM wakeup time. About an hour or more before 7:00 AM, your body has actually begun reheating itself, that is, your body temperature is beginning to creep up after having fallen most of the night. Therefore, if you awaken at seven o'clock with or without an alarm, you are engaging in a pattern very consistent with the body's desire to wake up.

Making this wake-up time consistent, combined with the fundamental sleep hygiene principle to use the bedroom only for sleep, leads to a direct challenge you must face each morning. When seven o'clock arrives, you must get up out of bed as soon as is reasonably possible (preferably within ten minutes) and leave the bedroom once you've finished with the bathroom, dressing and so forth.

When you apply this scheduling technique, do not be discouraged if this regular wakeup time does not produce an immediate impact on your bedtime. Given a fair trial and notwithstanding the old adage, don't be surprised to discover that the tail can indeed wag the dog.

10

Adding More Quality to Your Sleep

QUICK GUIDE

Problem: You want to sleep eight hours per night, but you only appear to be getting six.

Cause: Your focus on sleep quantity persuades you to believe the actual number of hours slept will determine how well you will feel in the morning.

Solution: Re-evaluate your expectations so you can improve sleep quality first and let quantity take care of itself.

A regular morning wakeup time coupled to a quick exit from the bedroom sends a very powerful sleep hygiene message to the brain. You are letting your mind know two things. First, wakefulness is separated from sleep because you've adopted the up and at 'em mindset. Second, you linked your wakefulness to the body's natural biological timekeeper, which works to get you up anyway.

In time, often in just a matter of days, this regular wakeup schedule stabilizes your bedtime, again for the same two reasons: 1) your body's circadian rhythm now starts winding down earlier in the nighttime; and 2) you've been out of bed all day keeping wakefulness separate from sleepiness.

If you do not get sleepy near to when you deem your proper bedtime, then we need to explore this issue. Say, for example, you wake up at seven o'clock and expect to go to bed by eleven at night to gain the standard eight hours of sleep.

Is this realistic?

Maybe, maybe not.

The more appropriate question to ask first is what is the average number of hours of sleep you think you're getting currently?

If you know you're only getting six or seven hours, then you might pose the question: "how realistic is it to think I might suddenly jump back up to eight?"

This question leads us back to the same quantity vs. quality issues, to which we typically declare:

If your average sleep is now six hours, then learning to capitalize on SIX GOOD HOURS OF SLEEP is the goal at hand.

Slowly, over time, perhaps these six extend to more hours while quality is maintained. But attempting the reverse, by adding quantity initially, often diminishes quality. This focus on quality for the chronic insomniac, sooner and later, proves more important than sleep quantity.

Add quality to your sleep first!

If your attempt at stabilizing the bedtime remains inconsistent, then we must examine your expectations about the total amount of sleep you believe you need. When you honestly and accurately ballpark your average total sleep time in this early phase of change, your goal is to spend only a bit more time in bed than the estimated sleep hours.

For instance, if you're now averaging six hours of sleep, you can add about thirty to sixty minutes to this total to come up with six and a half or seven hours of total time in bed. If you select seven hours of total bedtime, and your wakeup time is 7:00 AM, then bedtime would be midnight.

This bedtime might seem late if you've been trying for lights out at ten o'clock. But, with an average of only six hours of slumber, you are likely fragmenting your sleep by confusing your mind and body with a prolonged amount of time in bed.

To summarize, you must determine the average amount of sleep you're now getting and then add about thirty to sixty minutes to this total to arrive at total time in bed. This calculation assists you in determining a proper bed and wakeup time. If you extend your time in bed beyond this framework, your sleep becomes very inefficient, which brings us to the concept of sleep efficiency, a very practical way to attempt to improve sleep quality.

11

SLEEP PRESSURE INCREASES SLEEP EFFICIENCY

QUICK GUIDE

Problem: Your sleep efficiency is poor. The time you spend in bed notably exceeds the amount you spend asleep.

Cause: Your biological sleep pressure decreased as your habits blurred normal distinctions between sleep and waking behaviors.

Solution: Consider *limiting* your total sleep time so you never spend more than one-half hour awake in bed.

Did you know the longer you remain awake, the greater your physiological drive for sleep? This concept is known as *sleep pressure*. In other words, pressure to sleep builds up in our body as our time awake increases. Certainly, this point makes sense, but did you also know by increasing your sleep pressure, you can deepen your sleep as well? How then can an insomniac take advantage of this natural physiological response? The answer is to learn to apply sleep pressure to increase your *sleep efficiency*.

Sleep efficiency is your total sleep time (e.g. 9 hours) divided by your time in bed (e.g. 10 hours). These numbers are not equal as you must spend some time awake in bed, if only a few minutes when you first lie down, or the time between awakening and getting up. Time in bed therefore is always longer than time asleep. In the above example, your sleep efficiency would equal 90% (9/10).

Most normal adult sleepers will demonstrate 85% efficiency (6.75 hours of sleep/8 hours in bed) in the sleep lab, and usually higher levels such as 90% (7.25 hours sleep/8 hours in bed) at home. Many normal sleepers of all ages can achieve 95 to 99%; and yes, we'd love to be blessed with their genes! Children often sleep the highest efficiencies, regularly reaching 95%+ efficiency (9.50+ hours sleep/10 hours in bed).

Most insomniacs do not achieve these sleep efficiency percentages due to two fundamental problems. First, if you develop unrealistic expectations about falling asleep without being sleepy, then your total time in bed will increase as you lie awake in bed. Second, because so many insomniacs suffer from light or interrupted sleep, the tendency to wake up at least once (if not many times) during the night leads to lying awake in bed.

Talk of sleep pressure and efficiency returns us inevitably to sleep quality. As you increase sleep pressure, not only will efficiency increase, but overall quality goes up as well, because you restore some of your natural deep sleep. This improvement in quality can be realized in a matter of days (if not the very first night) by either shortening your time in bed, or by marginally restricting your amount of actual sleep.

Nearly everyone recognizes the concept of sleep pressure seems paradoxical to an insomniac if getting too little sleep is already a concern. It's a sensible concern, because most poor sleepers do indeed receive insufficient sleep; why, then, would you want to consider getting even less?

While it seems like harsh punishment to an insomniac, the fact is you already suffer an actual decrease in the total number of hours slept due to fragmented slumber. This light or disrupted sleep is nearly universal among insomniacs. If increasing your sleep pressure yields deeper and more qualitatively restful sleep, the number of hours slept proves irrelevant compared with the immediate and real gains from improved sleep quality.

Sometimes, only minor changes in your schedule need adjusting to increase natural sleep pressure and resulting deeper quality slumber. The two-for-one is you'll likely feel sleepy at the next bedtime and gain a huge boost in confidence! When you regain your natural desire to let yourself fall asleep at the appropriate time of your day-night cycle, you no longer plan or worry or obsess about your sleeping habits. Then, your whole process of sleeping runs its natural course like earlier in your life when sleep was a pleasure.

By temporarily producing a slight increase in sleep pressure, you foster better quality; and, over time, you may be able to expand your routine to a longer time in bed without sacrificing this quality. Once your mind and body integrate these elements into your schedule, your sleep has a much greater opportunity to return to a more natural cycle, which may lead to longer sleep coupled with higher quality.

An overarching key to success is learning to apply the sleep hygiene principle of separating sleeping behavior from waking behavior.

12

A Great Mattress Will
Not Last Forever

QUICK GUIDE

Problem: You do not sleep well on your current mattress.

Cause: Your mattress may be old and uncomfortable, but the larger problem is you developed a conditioned mistrust for your bedding, all but guaranteeing a poor night's sleep.

Solution: Buy a new mattress or improve your current one with supplemental foam pads and mattress covers.

We focused on the core sleep hygiene principles that must be addressed by essentially all who suffer from insomnia. At the heart of these principles is the singular distinction of learning to separate your sleep from your waking behaviors

You now appreciate how seemingly minor conditions may

provoke poor sleep by serving as major obstacles to your natural tendencies for sound slumber. Clock-watching is one example of a seemingly innocuous activity; yet, one that generates an outsized negative impact on your sleep. Some people have literally cured their insomnia by removing the clock or turning it to face the wall.

This classic example is the epitome of a tiny obstacle knocking you off course as you head down the road to better sleep. Often, such a tiny obstacle is present for months or years before you clearly see how it disturbs your sleep. It's akin to an old splinter under your skin causing constant irritation long before you might remove it. With this in mind, let's review several additional so-called minor conditions that may be interfering with your sleep.

Your mattress is an unsurprising example. Many people use a mattress for ten to twenty years partially because that's how they are advertised, but also it is more expedient (and less expensive) to keep using it. Good mattresses are not cheap and spending money to replace an old one does not appear convincingly cost-effective . . . at the moment.

How important is having the right mattress?

Let's ask another way. Would you be comfortable sleeping on a hardwood floor? a lumpy sofa? or a short pile rug?

Probably not. Yet, when was the last time you investigated the condition, texture, support and comfort of your current mattress?

Your sleep is intimately and obviously connected to your mattress. But, more importantly, if you develop mistrust about the quality and comfort of your bedding, can you imagine how readily this filters into your unconscious? Conversely, imagine the positive influence of looking forward to lying down on a mattress you know to be exceptionally comfortable.

Once again, we return to this process of connections. In this instance, it's not just that a mattress may be uncomfortable; it is more about your awareness of this discomfort setting you up night after night to expect poor quality or otherwise inadequate sleep. This relationship is so strong that were you to use a substandard mattress, but someone told you it was a great mattress, there is some chance your sleep would improve for at least the first night.

How do you determine if you have the right mattress? The answers will prove forthcoming once you become curious about whether or not your mattress is helping your sleep. If you're serious about upgrading, spend a few hours shopping at mattress stores. First, however, you must spend a good ten minutes or so lying on your own bed to test the comfort of your mattress. During this time, it will be helpful to let your thoughts drift a bit so any feelings of discomfort can surface in your mind. These thoughts and feelings inform you of how much you believe your mattress can or cannot affect your sleep, and they set the stage for making comparisons to other mattresses.

If you own a good mattress and you're convinced it's not the problem, there is no need to purchase another one. If you are suspicious, but not sure, you certainly need to confer with your bedmate. Once you gain a strong sense of what you may or may not like about your current bedding, then you need to visit mattress shops to test the vast array of options in the marketplace.

How much to pay for bedding depends on how much you can stretch for what you like. A mattress with a guarantee is worth it. Take your time to test mattresses, remember, go to just test! Sticker shock is normal; in my experience prices are set quite high so they can offer 50% off. Go to more than one store. Ask, "when is the seasonal sale?" Check prices online. You want to test out as many different styles as your time permits.

How high-tech do you want to go? Sleep medicine is becoming an enormous field; as such, more companies are investigating new and beneficial ways of improving the utility of mattresses and other bedding components. Air cushioning, a variety of foam materials as well as advances in traditional coil structures give you legitimate options.

As always, you get what you pay for. And, now the choices are so vast, you definitely don't want to buy right away. In addition to taking the time to have the manufacturer's warranty spelled out clearly, you also want to explore the most technological innovations. In particular, learn about technologies that control or influence temperatures. Some brands are now advertising how they remove heat to keep the bedding cooler. This particular area is likely to prove one of the most important innovations in building a better mattress.

13

THE ADVANTAGE OF A QUIET AND DARK BEDROOM

QUICK GUIDE

Problem: Excess light and noise disturb your sleep.

Cause: Environmental circumstances, for example, insensitive neighbors or other uncontrollable events, interfere with your sleep and worsen your insomnia.

Solution: Earplugs and nightshades should be a last resort. Talk with your neighbors while expecting to have to talk to them again . . . and again; do so candidly but without hostility: remember, if they don't have sleep problems, they do not understand your predicament. Be imaginative and consider a white noise device.

Would you knowingly try to fall asleep each night in a hot, brightly lit room with stale air, lots of dust, and loud, raucous music playing at your bedside?

Obviously not. To be sure, there are those who do not suffer from insomnia who can sleep like a log under such adverse conditions; but, for an insomniac, it would be putting out a fire with gasoline.

Your environment is another one of these seemingly minor conditions with profound consequences on your sleep if not attended to in a healthy manner.

Light, air, temperature, noise and cleanliness are crucial environmental factors, and each person must determine what works best. More critically, however, because many normal sleepers tend to be insensitive to those with poor sleep, these issues require the insomniac to develop assertiveness when other people or circumstances disturb the sleep environment.

A completely dark room is the best possible sleep environment based solely on the physiologic responses of the human body. Darkness does not account however for an individual's need to feel safe and secure in the bedroom. If a night light is required, that's fine.

Keep in mind, if you are willing to experiment with a darker room, you may reap the benefits of placing your body in synch with the natural day-night cycle that promotes sleep. And, opaque window shades are not so expensive. Last, if you want less light, but circumstances are beyond your control, most can learn to use night shades over the eyes.

Noise reduction, unfortunately, is a more complicated affair. First off, your last resort is earplugs, which only work up to a point unless you're willing to spend the money for custom fitted devices, although OTC foam plugs work well for many.

The problem of noise, however, is pervasive unless you live in a very rural environment, but then the chickens, pheasants, and other birds nab you early in the morning. This pervasive noise is so intense in our so-called modern society that most people rarely experience what a long time ago used to be called "quiet." It's possible some do not even know a state of quiet as a real thing. Were you living in an exceptionally well insulated home to shield you from outside noises, you still might notice your sleep disturbed by the inside rumblings from heating and cooling equipment, refrigerators and other appliances if you are very sensitive to noise as are many insomniacs.

Because good sleepers usually are able to sleep anywhere, they adapt to the din of traffic noises, or the roar of planes overhead, or sirens, or loud parties, or barking dogs or whatever. To many of these individuals, it is inconceivable noise could somehow hamper someone else's sleep. Some are so dense if you told them they were making too much noise in their neighboring apartment, their immediate reaction would be gross confusion, followed usually by some low-level hostility.

This attitude is problematic because in dealing with noise issues you're weighing in directly against the grain of society. In our over-stimulated environment, the majority of people allow their senses to deaden so they can adapt to both chronic low-grade noise as well as loud and raucous disturbances. There ought to be a law! In fact, there are many such laws on your side, but it is a delicate, if not touchy, encounter to assert your rights for a modicum of quiet.

I could recount numerous stories of both friends and patients where the cure proved worse than the disease, so hostile and upsetting was the response from their noisy neighbors. These insensitive responses led to more frustration and subsequently worse sleep from the build up of unvented irritation. And, all that they had asked was for someone to simply turn down the volume.

Consider the possibility of honest discussion by offering to explain your difficulty with insomnia, but be prepared to lie, yes lie, or say anything to convince them of your need to sleep on a regular schedule. Tell them you get ear infections when you wear earplugs; tell them you're in school and you have to take a special exam every morning in class; tell them you're working eighty hours per week and you only get a chance to sleep five or six hours a night; tell them anything! They may or may not listen. You might also consider a mediation service, but then you would have to convince your neighbor to enter into such an arrangement.

When all else fails, seriously consider the concept of white noise and the new array of other noise machines, or simply listening to the sounds of rain on your phone. Although some insomniacs find this method irritating, others gain genuine relief with a well-placed fan or some other soothing sound-making device. Noise cancelling is usually less irritating than earplugs and certainly better than having to deal with the anticipation of your neighbors or the surrounding communities incessant attacks on your eardrums.

If earplugs are your last resort, go for the 33-decibel foam version; they can prove very effective short or long-term.

14

FIND THE PROPER BEDROOM TEMPERATURE

QUICK GUIDE

Problem: You want to sleep in fresh, clean air from an open window, but you feel more comfortable in a warm bedroom.

Cause: Insomniacs may feel chilly at bedtime because their skin temperature may be lower than normal.

Solution: Experiment with the proper mix of blankets, a fan and a cracked window. Consider a hot bath before bedtime. Aim for the fresh air approach, but defer to your need for a warm environment in the first portion of the night.

———————

From light and noise, we move on to fresh air, temperature and cleanliness.

A clean sleeping environment has two major benefits for you, one physical, the other mental. From a health standpoint, a clean bedroom will promote healthier breathing while you sleep. The build up of dust, mites, molds and other allergens and irritants in the room, or worse in your bedding, will cause sneezing, coughing, and nasal congestion.

To sleep well, you need to breathe well through your nose.

Cleanliness requires regular dusting and vacuuming as well as frequent linen changes. More so, a mattress cover definitely serves as a barrier to particulate matter harbored inside the mattress itself. Whether or not you need to explore hypoallergenic pillows or other specialized bedding is a matter of cost and personal preference.

Regardless of how you approach things, it is essential to feel a sense of comfort about sleeping in a clean bedroom. A dusty room irritating your nose delivers a strong message to the brain heralding the onset of compromised breathing while you sleep. Thus, the mental aspect of sleeping in an unclean room eventually produces an association significant enough to prevent or disrupt your slumber.

Another consideration is the need for fresh air. Many people sleep with an open or cracked window all year long regardless of weather. Notwithstanding the possibility of greater exposure to allergens such as pollens, fresh air can promote a sense of cleanliness and thereby facilitate easier breathing.

While sleeping, it is useful to recognize your body enters into a catabolic state, that is, because you are no longer eating or drinking, your metabolism shifts to a different mechanism for producing energy to keep your organ systems functioning. This mechanism involves ketosis or the breakdown of stored fats in lieu of your daily dietary intake. Ketosis along with an individual's propensity for sweating while sleeping can produce strong odors noticeable upon awakening. The staleness of these odors can be removed while (or after) sleeping if you crack a window or use a fan with an open bedroom door.

Leaving the bedroom window open affects the temperature of the room, which is a major consideration for virtually all sleepers. The variability here is enormous as some people sleep more comfortably when the thermometer drops *below* 60 degrees Fahrenheit whereas others prefer 70 degrees or *above*. Scientific studies have not been able to demonstrate conclusively an ideal sleeping temperature, although research does lean in support of a cooler environment. However, this information adds little to *your* sleep if you developed a preference for a warmer environment.

If your insomnia is exacerbated by a painful condition such as arthritis or low back problems, then a cooler environment could make sleep worse. Moreover, many insomniacs suffer from a type of physical tenseness producing vasoconstriction (tightening) of the blood vessels in the skin. Blood flow decreases and creates a chilly feeling in the hands and feet of the insomniac. As such, when going to bed the insomniac feels cool and may require additional blankets.

Complicating matters, a few hours later an insomniac often relaxes leading to vasodilation of these same vessels, and then the individual wakes up feeling too warm. As you can imagine, the sheets or blankets now need to be pulled back. This cycling during the night in some insomniacs proves quite frustrating and may require more advanced technology such as mattress temperature innovations to solve in a seamless fashion.

Finding the right combination with fresh air, appropriate blankets and a quiet fan is usually worth the effort. If, however, you sleep in the same room with someone else who has different fresh air and temperature requirements, you may need to be more adaptable. If the environment feels too cold, then a hot shower before bedtime can work magic. Or, if the room is too hot, a lukewarm bath or shower can dissipate some of the heat off of your body surface to cool you down. Again, the use of blankets and a quiet fan for your side of the bed can also make a difference.

15

EAT RIGHT, SLEEP RIGHT

QUICK GUIDE

Problem: Your diet affects your sleep.

Cause: Heavy meals at bedtime promote indigestion, and poor diets in general lead to poor health and bad sleep.

Solution: Never eat a large meal close to bedtime and re-evaluate your diet to insure lots of fruits, vegetables and unprocessed foods, the foundation of any good regimen.

After you awaken in the morning, all your ensuing daily activities could impact your next night's rest. The very first activity of getting up and out of bed fairly quickly is a prime factor in teaching you to mentally and physically separate your sleep from your waking periods.

Many other waking factors also enhance or limit your capacity for sleep, including your diet, mealtimes, use of alcohol, cigarettes and caffeine, your sex and exercise habits, your propensity for napping, and finally your style of handling worries and stress throughout the day.

A healthy diet promotes a positive influence on your sleep, just as an unhealthy diet yields a negative one. A healthy diet for most people consists of a lot of fruits and vegetables along with a variety of whole grains and certain dairy products and animal proteins. A balanced diet of this sort provides a solid nutritional base for your body's metabolism that, in turn, adds to your ability to remain fit and healthy.

In contrast, foods triggering constipation, reflux or other forms of indigestion not only impair your health during the daytime but also cause insomnia at night, including both difficulties in falling asleep or waking throughout the night.

Moreover, there is clear evidence a poor or unbalanced diet leads to worse health, inducing more infections such as colds or flu, or more aches and pains from muscle strains and cramps. At the most fundamental level, if your diet is poor and your health suffers, you can expect any number of minor ailments to interfere with your sleep, whether it's a cold that interferes with your breathing, a backache that awakens you when you roll over in bed or indigestion that prevents the onset of sleep.

Eating at regular times also aids your sleep on two counts. First, it promotes consistency, keeping you in synch with your natural biological rhythm. Second, if you maintain a schedule for your last meal of the day at a time not too late in the evening, then your digestion is less likely to interfere with your sleep. Large or heavy meals eaten within a couple of hours of bedtime promote gastric distress throughout the night, notably esophageal reflux where the digestive juices back up from the stomach into the esophagus to cause heartburn.

While consistency and timing benefit sleep, nothing compares to the larger dietary issue affecting most people, namely, what to eat? Too many believe we "live to eat," but as we mature, we realize we "eat to live." Learning first to avoid foods that provide no health benefits is the smartest dietary strategy to follow for your health and your sleep.

You may also experiment with specific foods in a targeted manner to promote better sleep. Foods higher in L-tryptophan may aid some people's slumber although the scientific evidence for this remains incomplete. Still, some insomniacs report success with a turkey sandwich or a baked sweet potato as a late evening snack. Other sources of naturally occurring L-tryptophan can be considered as well.

The supplement version is back on the market after a shocking episode in the late 1980s where a condition known as eosinophilic-myalgia syndrome (EMS) developed in some L-tryptophan users. Investigations into the link were initially thought related to a contaminant in the supplement. Nonetheless, some reports still link EMS to L-tryptophan while noting it is a rare occurrence. Obviously, caution is advised.

Whether or not other supplements, including, theanine, tyrosine, calcium and magnesium have a role in improving sleep remains unproven even though many nutrition-oriented stores would be delighted to have you believe otherwise. On the other hand, if you take an investigative approach, enjoy perusing health magazines, and feel comfortable using nutritional supplements, it may be reasonable to pursue such a path. While certain benefits have yet to be clearly proven regarding supplemental vitamins and other nutrients, it is also clear that scientific research into these areas is quite limited. Therefore, the medical-scientific community may be uninformed, perhaps even misguided, about alternative approaches to these health issues.

Finally, well into the 21st century we find an abundance of over-the-counter supplements, vitamins, minerals, herbs and other concoctions advertised as sleep aids. I am a great believer in the free enterprise system, and the good news is some products actually improve sleep. More good news is found in the USA and many other countries where you are allowed to make your own judgments on whether or not to purchase these sleep aids and conduct your own do-it-yourself experiments.

It is of course at your own risk that you choose to do so, and regrettably, the scientific community does not put much emphasis on testing these products. Which means you are likely relying on advertising programs, testimonials or word of mouth in making your decisions. Theoretically, these pathways could prove relevant, because you would be the first person to know whether the product is working for you or not.

I am persuaded that several compounds yield sleep benefits, but I do not recommend specific items as it is crystal clear you need to figure out what works for you, and equally important you are the one who will need to monitor for any harmful side-effects.

In sum, I strongly encourage this over-the-counter approach compared to the well-know side effects of most prescription sleeping pills.

16

ALCOHOL, CAFFEINE AND NICOTINE

QUICK GUIDE

Problem: Your use of alcohol, caffeine and nicotine are interfering with sleep.

Cause: All three substances interfere with either your ability to fall asleep or stay asleep by producing mini-withdrawal states.

Solution: Reduce or refrain from using these drugs altogether or at least after dinner. Caffeine may require an earlier stopping time; nicotine may permit a later one.

Alcohol, nicotine and caffeine ought to be a proverbial no-brainer when it comes to sleep, yet these drugs are so commonplace that it is unusual to meet someone who doesn't use any of them. Moreover, there are many people who use these drugs and sleep fine; therefore, the real issue is how each substance might affect an insomniac.

Nicotine has the most subtle impact by affecting your breathing over time. In the short run, if you smoke close to bedtime, you may temporarily stimulate yourself, then experience a mild nicotine withdrawal state throughout the night. In this withdrawal, the body craves another dose of nicotine, but most wait until the morning to receive it. This could lead to restless sleep and some awakenings.

Alcohol's impact is more insidious than nicotine because it actually sedates you and promotes deep sleep in the early portion of your slumber. But, like nicotine, when the alcohol wears off by the middle of the night or earlier, a mini-withdrawal state occurs, yielding a definite lightening of your sleep. In other words, while alcohol could help to induce sleep, it will create difficulties in remaining asleep. It is not uncommon for someone who drinks near bedtime to arouse in the middle of the night and not to return to sleep.

In these situations, there are those who drink again to go back to sleep. If you did not know this previously, let me be crystal clear: drinking alcoholic beverages in the middle of the night to get sleepy again unquestionably places you at high risk for the problem of alcoholism. Find another solution, please!

Even so, many adults drink 1 or 2 glasses of wine in the evening to relax. They welcome this very human behavior to wash away stress and worries without any impulse to abuse alcohol. Thus, some insomniacs could use this small amount of wine to start winding down well before bedtime.

Caffeine acts as a stimulant and a highly effective one in a variety of situations. Its use close to bedtime could produce a very attentive state and serve as an undesirable obstacle to falling asleep. Caffeine is usually served in four categories of beverages and food: coffee, tea, sodas and chocolate. The amount of caffeine varies in each one, but all possess sufficient levels to disturb sleep. Once again, a mini-withdrawal state could occur in the middle of the night if you are a chronic caffeine user.

Summing up, alcohol and caffeine are widely used in society and serve many purposes, healthy and unhealthy. Abusing alcohol actually damages your throat and increases your risk for sleep apnea, yet when used in moderation may aid your coping with daily stress. Caffeine offers great potential to enhance daytime alertness and energy, which improves the quality of your life at work, home or play. As long as you can minimize the caffeine dosage, perhaps experimenting with green or white tea, then you only need to gauge how early in the day to cease use of caffeinated beverages. Your goal is to maximize benefits while preventing too much caffeine running through your system near bedtime. Tracking data about when and how much alcohol or caffeine you consume could lead to a better understanding of their impact on your sleep and how to fine tune your efforts.

17

SEX AND EXERCISE

QUICK GUIDE

Problem: Exercise is not helping your sleep.

Cause: If you engage in exercise too late in the day, its alerting influence may last beyond your normal bedtime.

Solution: Light exercise, such as walking in the evening is fine, but heavier exertion should be reserved for earlier in the day and preferably before dinner.

———

Physical activity generates a noticeable impact on your sleep propensity. You may remember a time at a younger age when vigorous physical exertion during the daytime led to solid sleep at night.

Most people benefit tremendously by engaging in significant physical exercise every day and ideally for much longer than generally prescribed. Certainly, gaining aerobic capacity (e.g. running) or engaging in extended moderate activity (e.g. walking) provides healthy results.

The real issue with respect to health in general and sleep in particular is the innate need of humans to be physically active. To think otherwise goes against the grain of human history except for the last few sedentary decades of the twentieth century up to the present day. People are built to do things, whether physical labor, doing chores, making repairs, traipsing up and down steps, walking/jogging to the corner market and so on.

In modern times, extended activities like hiking, endurance swimming, lengthy walks, or even golf (no electric carts, please) encourage you to use your body over a period of time that more closely matches what your level of activity might have been years ago no matter where you lived. Perhaps one day our society will evolve to recapture this lost emphasis on physicality. If so, the norm will be to engage in physical activities throughout various portions of the day, some perhaps related to work, others to play.

Nowadays, exercise often gets blocked off into predetermined segments of your life. You may jog in the morning or walk in the evening. Certainly, something is better than nothing, but because you become accustomed to only one portion of the day to exert yourself, the timing of this exercise may produce an undesirable outcome. For example, if you run aerobically or lift weights later in the evening, say a few hours before bedtime, the aftereffect may actually alert you and inhibit your ability to fall asleep. Conversely, if you exercise late in the afternoon before dinner, the immediate overheating of your body through physical exertion may promote a steeper decline of your body temperature near bedtime and thus promote sleepiness.

In summary, some exercise is better than none, but timing may prove pivotal in determining the response. And, whenever possible, more periods of exercise should be adopted, like running in the morning, walking after lunch, and gardening in the early evening.

One short update based on only one study: newer research suggests late evening resistance-type exercise may promote deeper sleep.

———

Timing of sexual activity also yields distinctly different effects usually specific to each person, and for which almost nothing is written about with regards to sleep.

Though we emphasized the use of the bedroom only for sleep, this point is not meant to preclude or hamper your sex life in anyway. In fact, in terms of associations described for most sleep hygiene steps, sex and sleep are inextricably linked. After all, most sexual encounters for the vast majority of individuals occur at night, in bed and just prior to sleep. The second most common encounter would probably occur in the morning, in bed after waking up from sleep.

Your sex life, therefore, affects your sleep life. However, very little research is available to suggest what the impact might be. Moreover, in discussing with different people you'll discover a wide range of responses. For example, some people note sex or orgasm in particular, will always help them fall asleep, while others declare the exact opposite, that is, sex alerts them so much they can no longer fall asleep. This range of opinions is expressed by both men and women.

Thus, responses to both exercise and sex can be different for different people, yet there is no question our bodies were made to engage in physical activity and love-making. Interestingly, both experiences lead to considerable reduction in physical tension; and this tension is believed to be one of the leading physical contributors to chronic insomnia. Sometimes the phrase, "somatized tension," is used to describe the presence of physical tightness of various muscle groups in the insomniac.

"Somatic" indicates how a human unknowingly lets things fester in the body to produce a state of tension. Things could include thoughts, worries, feelings, sensations, and stressors clinging to your body as unhealthy pent-up energy. Generally, this somatized tension does not find a release, and the result is sleeplessness.

Learning to appreciate how exercise and sex reduce pent-up energy as well as how essential coping skills play a key function in emotional processing may directly improve your insomnia.

18

MAKE NAPS SHORT AND EARLY

QUICK GUIDE

Problem: Napping during the day feels good, yet it seems to be affecting nighttime sleep.

Cause: Naps too long or too late in the day will decrease your overall sleep pressure and thus cause problems at night.

Solution: Napping is fine if you accept you only need so much sleep every 24-hour period. Limit your nap to earlier in the day and to no more than thirty minutes, if not less.

The question of napping is raised by some insomniacs who are often puzzled by their ability to fall asleep during the daytime on some occasions, yet continue with difficulty falling asleep at night. There is nothing fundamentally wrong with napping, but it is necessary to appreciate and follow a few guidelines if you choose to nap so as to not interfere with your nighttime sleep.

Foremost, assume in the course of any 24-hour period you need only so much sleep; it could be eight hours, or it might only be six. If you choose to use up some sleep time during the day, that's all right, particularly if you feel refreshed after a nap, and it doesn't interfere with your nighttime sleep.

However, naps could interfere with your night time sleep in several ways. First, if you nap too late in the afternoon or early in the evening, your mind and body are not likely to be in the mood to fall asleep again at night. Second, if you nap for a long period, or take 2 or more shorter naps, amounting to more than an hour, a similar problem arises; namely, your mind and body already experienced sufficient sleep so now you're not ready to engage in sleep again for several more hours.

The later or the longer you nap creates more potential for this behavior to become self-defeating regarding nighttime efforts. You may find yourself staying up well past midnight before genuine sleepiness reappears to lead you naturally toward a good night's slumber.

Why nap at all then?

Harvey Penick, the famous golf instructor was fond of saying, "if I ask you to take an aspirin, don't take the whole bottle." The same goes for napping. If you use a short, refreshing catnap (< 20 - 30 min) early rather than late in the day, it's doubtful such a sleep period would interfere with nighttime sleep. For some, 2 – 10 min naps work wonders to regain daytime alertness and energy.

Sleep specialists believe your ability to nap in such a manner builds confidence in your overall ability to fall asleep and thus enhances your attempt at night.

Moreover, napping is common in many cultures; often, a lengthy nap period at midday and a shorter nighttime sleep period are the standard. One reason for splitting your sleep into two distinct time periods may be explained by our natural biological clock, known as the circadian rhythm. At night, through the release of melatonin, the circadian rhythm shifts towards a lower body temperature, which promotes falling and staying asleep.

A similar though less noticeable temperature drop may occur during the daytime for a much briefer time span. Around or just after lunchtime, the body's temperature can level off or briefly decline. This time period may last a few minutes to a few hours, but some degree of sleepiness is produced in virtually anyone.

Caffeine of course masks this reflex; but notwithstanding the use of stimulants like coffee, many could easily adopt a system to nap or embrace a *siesta* in synchrony with this short, natural change in body temperature. This change should be coupled with an expectation for a shorter nighttime sleep period. Then again, such a schedule must realistically fit in with your work and home life in which case the benefits of a short nap clearly outweigh any disadvantages, inconveniences or conflicts.

As you can imagine, there are reasons it may seem easier to feel sleepy during the day and to actually nod off for several minutes or even a couple of hours; however, to reiterate you probably need only so much sleep in the course of any 24-hour period. If you sleep too much during the day, then you remove or reduce your natural physiological sleep pressure that could have served you well that night.

Remember, *most people build sleep pressure by staying awake.* Notwithstanding, if you suffer from a psychiatric illness such as manic-depression, then shortening your sleep length can trigger a manic episode. As relevant, this information should be discussed with your psychiatrist.

More generally, even if you enjoy a lengthy nap, it certainly could decrease sleep pressure followed by difficulty falling out that night. Then, a new cycle of insomnia might be triggered.

Overall, it is also helpful to evaluate the basic psychology of falling asleep during the day. The feeling of sleepiness sometimes occurs as a response to a boring or difficult emotional situation. If you have trouble falling asleep at night, but notice a much easier propensity for doing so during the day while attending a boring lecture or meeting in the early afternoon, then we usually believe it's time to ask yourself three distinct questions.

First, is the sleepiness the result of sleep deprivation? Even when you've improved your sleep quality, each person still needs a relatively set number of hours of sleep. By fixing sleep quality, it's usually easier to calculate how many hours you need. So, if you think you're not getting enough, then you have a straightforward explanation for why you want to nap during the day.

Second, what if your sleep quality is not as high as it should be? What if you are suffering subtle sleep fragmentation during the night for which you have no awareness? This problem is one of the most common causes for napping during the daytime.

And, third, as above, what if the dilemma is not really about sleep? The feeling of sleepiness is a perfect defense against people, situations, or circumstances you wish to escape from, if only temporarily. People really can get very sleepy in the face of unpleasant business or chores or relationship issues they would prefer to avoid.

Finally, there is the possibility of boredom. True boredom is a wonderful thing if your goal is to fall asleep. Many an insomniac wishes she could recreate a genuine boring state around bedtime, because the chances for falling asleep would be so much higher.

Many sleep professionals preach the necessity to avoid all types of stimulation close to bedtime. This stance refers to TV, radio, internet, etc. that you find stimulating or aggravating. The same holds for what goes on in your mind; can you put aside thoughts, feelings or images that are only going to vex you when you'd rather be sleeping?

With respect to disturbing emotions, there is no question some individuals escape from unpleasant feelings by becoming sleepy and/or falling asleep. This behavior can be quite healthy, particularly for your nighttime sleep as it may yield a necessary breather from emotional turmoil, which after a good night of slumber might sort itself out, perhaps through the wonders of dreaming.

With respect to napping, however, if you discover your sleepy feeling is preceded by some problematic emotional conflict, a nap could be postponing your need to directly confront these feelings. In this case, despite noticing little difficulty falling asleep after lunch, bedtime might become an issue as you compounded the problem of insomnia by using up some of your natural sleep pressure with this nap.

To nap or not to nap has subtle wrinkles that must be ironed out so it is clear why and how short daytime sleep periods may be beneficial or harmful to your nighttime sleep.

Now let's return to more general questions about how emotions, stress, and managing one's feelings have an effect on your sleep. We've mentioned a few tips in relationship to napping, which serves as a starting point. We'll delve deeper to see how your mood and your emotions dramatically impact your complete sleep cycle.

19

Stop Worrying and Start Sleeping

QUICK GUIDE

Problem: Mental attitudes and emotional worries are disrupting your sleep.

Cause: Worries and other negative emotions produce negative thoughts and feelings that keep you awake in bed fretting about your problems.

Solution: Consider a short worry session earlier in the day to focus on your conflicts at a time unrelated to sleep. Also consider the help of a friend or perhaps a mental health professional to teach you successful psychological coping skills to improve the way you handle stress.

Your mental attitude prior to bedtime has a great, perhaps the greatest, influence on your capacity to sleep soundly. This attitude may include: state of relaxation, body tension, anxieties and worries, and overall mental health.

Mental health is an on-going process filtering into every part of your life. For example, tension in the body does not suddenly arise a few minutes before bedtime; rather, it usually builds throughout the day and eventually causes an inability to relax sufficiently to fall asleep.

Dealing with mental health issues is not something to put off. Learning to recognize tension in the body and learning how to relax can be worked on throughout the day. Meditation, yoga, deep breathing, imagery work, and light physical exercise are a few techniques to relax. It may prove especially helpful to engage in relaxing behavior in the evening as you wind down toward bedtime.

Physical tension or the inability to relax stems from unresolved emotional conflicts or problems. People who have difficulty sleeping often discover the source of their tension is pent-up feelings such as fear, sadness, guilt, anger or frustration. Others notice ill-defined feelings such as anxiety.

Learning to pinpoint these emotions is a necessary first step in improving your mental health. The more these feelings are avoided, denied or suppressed, the more likely to fester inside your mind-body. A prime example could be someone suffering from insomnia, who doesn't realize his or her inability to fall asleep is a red flag signaling emotional distress about some issue, conflict, relationship, etc. The longer one avoids the warning, the more likely the insomnia will continue, if not worsen. Sometimes, the insomnia is a harbinger of depression, which could develop in a few months or more than a year after the start of the sleeplessness.

The single most consistently destructive emotional state that affects our sleep revolves around anticipated problems: in short, our worries. Worrying about the future is one of the surest paths to insomnia!

On a rational level, it is of some benefit to appreciate **how worrying rarely solves the problem worried about**.

If you allow yourself to recognize worries only beget more worries, you may want to explore what some call worry sessions. At a point earlier in the day (no later than after dinner), some find it useful to focus their anxieties into a single short session (through self-talk or pad and paper) with the understanding that once the time is over (say, ten to twenty minutes), no further worrying is permitted. Specifically, you commit to avoid being held hostage by fretful thoughts. While such an approach may be appealing, some people's anxieties may get the best of them and simply initiate a cascading process that knows no end.

It is certainly natural and common to experience some anxiety during the day; however, the feeling of anxiety is often a mask for another even stronger emotion, usually more threatening than so-called worrying. For example, if you identify a work situation where you are very *angry* at your boss while simultaneously *fearful* of losing your job if you express this anger, the mind's natural defenses typically prevail to cloud these specific issues.

Why would your mind cooperate with this attempt at self-deception? Simply, if you expressed your genuine anger, perhaps your boss would dismiss you. Instead, the better part of valor would be to bite your tongue but then anxiety is sure to follow in such situations unless you develop the skill of learning to recognize and appreciate the depths of your anger and fear without having to act on them in a way that might jeopardize your job.

Some individuals' emotional distress requires professional help. A poor sleeper may develop the belief that if she could only sleep better, then her bad feelings would disappear. In fact, many people feel they are depressed because of poor sleep. This view may be accurate, but it is more likely a two-way street: depression may induce or worsen poor sleep, while poor sleep might induce or worsen depression.

The relationship between mental health and sleep is not always straightforward. Talking with your physician, a mental health professional, a clergyman or a close friend about emotional problems may be one of the most successful strategies you can use to improve your sleep. If your particular style of handling (or mishandling) worries and stress is a major contributor to your sleeplessness, then a mental health professional, in just a few short sessions, may be able to teach you a different coping style that will also improve your problems with insomnia.

If you are unsure how to connect the dots between your sleep issues and mental health problems, I encourage you to grab a copy of my book, *Life Saving Sleep: New Horizons in Mental Health Treatment*, where you will find six chapters addressing how anxiety and other emotions play havoc with your sleep. In the book, you'll learn advanced techniques to directly work through your difficult emotions, which prove to be some of the most potent treatments for chronic insomnia.

Last, bedtime prayers are potent. Most realize their value, because the themes and specific details address vexing difficulties in our waking lives. Prayer is certainly worth daily practice and may provide great comfort at bedtime.

20

BEYOND SLEEP HYGIENE

QUICK GUIDE

Problem: Sleep hygiene has helped to reduce but not eliminate your problems with insomnia.

Cause: There are many different types of insomnia, most of which benefit from the applications of sleep hygiene, but many require additional measures.

Solution: Consider seeking help from a sleep specialist to help you uncover physical sleep disorders that might be a deeper cause for your sleeplessness.

———

Sleep ought to be a natural process occurring without significant effort. **You let yourself fall asleep.**

Why a person loses this natural ability is often related to several items we've addressed regarding sleep hygiene. Sleep hygiene is a simple set of guidelines that will help you to appreciate what was hopefully at one point in your earlier life a very natural process. By following these guidelines, you give yourself the opportunity to recapture the natural feeling that enhanced your ability to fall asleep and stay asleep. Moreover, advanced sleep hygiene guidelines provide you with some flexibility and allow for individual adaptation. Incorporating these principles into your waking and sleeping habits is often an effective way to improve your sleep.

But now the question arises: what if these steps turn out to be only half the picture…or worse less than half?

Fast Asleep was written for the vast majority of mild to moderate insomniacs whose difficulties usually respond to the straightforward cognitive-behavioral changes suggested through the principles and practice of advanced sleep hygiene. Even among those with more complex forms of insomnia, sleep hygiene offers some hope and yields some improvement.

But a substantial number of individuals with complex insomnia need more help. They may for example require the services of a sleep specialist to guide them through more exacting strategies such as sleep restriction therapy coupled with the use of extensive diary and journal exercises. In such instances, working with a professional trained in the subtleties and nuances of sleep medicine could enhance your level of success.

For those with persisting difficulties, I would like to leave you with two important considerations to guide you in your further quest of a cure.

First, it is imperative to recognize insomnia is often a problem caused by several things, not just one thing; yet, like a jigsaw puzzle, you must start with one piece. As you join more pieces of this puzzle together, a picture begins to form. However, it proves frustrating and overwhelming if you are routinely selecting a part to the puzzle that doesn't fit.

Where to start your attack on the problem of sleeplessness might prove crucial to how fast you make headway. When you discover a key piece to your personal insomnia puzzle, many of the other parts fall naturally into place. It is for these reasons sleep hygiene often, but certainly not always, proves the very best program with which to initiate your exploration of your insomnia problem.

Thereafter, other factors are considered. And, among many insomniacs a piece often overlooked is sleep physiology as opposed to sleep psychology. Holistically speaking, mind-body medicine always considers the impact of both mental and physical components of health.

Which brings us to the second and perhaps most astonishing idea for your consideration. As indicated in the Preface and to close out this book, in my personal and professional experience, I have researched and learned from many insomniacs, who contrary to the current and prevailing scientific view from the field of sleep medicine, actually suffer from subtle sleep breathing and sleep movement disorders.

These disorders are not easy to diagnose because the current technology used to evaluate sleep is similar to the situation in which one would find oneself using a magnifying glass to search for something only observable with a microscope. New technology is emerging every year and soon, I predict, it will become clearer to our field of medicine, physical factors or disorders are a much greater contributor to insomnia than has been previously recognized.

The wonderful thing about this point is such technology will ultimately confirm what most doctors were taught and hopefully are still taught in medical school: **that the patient in some way or**

another always carries a special knowledge and understanding of their own problem. Although this knowledge may not sound particularly scientific, it still provides explanations that physicians and scientists should never forget to acknowledge *and* utilize for patients' benefit.

In the instance of sleep problems, patients have long offered the following refrain: "doctor, if I could just sleep better, I'm sure my depression would improve." To this refrain, many patients receive an equally resounding chorus from their doctors that goes something like this: "actually, if we just treated your depression, I bet your sleep problems would get better, too." Both doctor and patient are probably on the right track, but I predict with the advent of greater technological sophistication, we will see how treatment of subtle sleep breathing and sleep movement disorders cures a much larger number of insomniacs than most sleep specialists, let alone doctors, would have expected based on our current understanding of sleep medicine. And, treating sleep-breathing conditions will likewise improve depression.

I offer this last bit of info for those of you who feel particularly frustrated in your quest for better sleep and feel in some ways your anguished cries for help have fallen on ears deafened by what appears to be a wax build-up of modern medicine. In time, I trust and hope for many of you, a closer inspection of these subtle sleep problems will remove the last remaining obstacles in your journey down the path to healthy sleep.

And, finally, writing 25 years later after a much earlier version of this book was published, my research teams published more than 30 peer-reviewed scientific publications proving sleep-disordered breathing is indeed joined at the hip in a huge number of chronic insomniacs, particularly those who have been failing drug therapies.

Twenty-five years ago, I finished this chapter "Good luck and sweet dreams!" Now, I can tell you the luck you need is the specific task of finding a knowledgeable sleep doctor who closely follows research and understands the critical links between sleep breathing and waking up in the middle of night.

If you find the right doc, I could almost guarantee your chances are terrific for finding those sweet dreams as well.

EPILOGUE

The field of sleep medicine must still be considered a relatively new, if not primitive field. We still know very little about the fundamental ways in which sleeping or dreaming affect our lives and health. We know sleep and dreams are important, but our ability to define and describe normal sleep and dreaming remains remarkably limited.

Insomnia is a sleep disorder of which a great deal of descriptive information has been gathered, but there is only a small amount of knowledge on the underlying mechanisms that cause or promote insomnia. Current emphasis remains on behavioral or psycho-physiological explanations for insomnia, which implicate one's attitude, beliefs, habits, and circumstances and possibly biological predisposition as causative factors.

This book therefore focused on advanced sleep hygiene, a program that features parts of the therapy known as cognitive-behavioral treatments for insomnia or CBT-I. And though a full course of CBT-I may prove curative in many insomnia cases, it remains puzzling how sleep medicine has failed to develop a definitive therapy that *consistently* and *completely* cures insomnia, particularly for those with the most severe sleep complaints.

In my opinion, sleep medicine has neglected to make greater

strides in the treatment of insomnia because it has tended to focus narrowly on two prevailing approaches. The first, as described, is the psychological aspect, which is often very helpful but typically not curative for moderate to severe insomnia.

The second is pharmacotherapy, that is, treatment with sedatives or anxiety-reducing drugs or antidepressants. While pharmacotherapy may be effective in some patients, drugs are rarely curative except in short-term cases, and they produce adverse effects. These adverse effects are not inconsequential and may include higher mortality rates among those who use sedatives on a nightly basis. More concerning is the use of multiple medications to treat the symptoms of broken sleep, and here again results are poor.

What then are the obstacles that might be preventing the field of sleep medicine from maximizing the therapeutic effects of insomnia treatments?

I believe the biggest obstacles are sleep clinicians' and sleep researchers' inability to think outside the box to appreciate how complaints of insomnia might actually be linked to a physical component. Instead, in their minds, insomnia can only be a problem in the patient's mind.

Unfortunately, so many physicians and therapists and others who treat insomnia automatically assume a patient stating, "there is something wrong with my sleep," or "I don't sleep very well," can only indicate mental dysfunction, which then is declared the cause of the problem. On the other hand, if I show up in the Emergency Department complaining my arm hurts and the x-ray says it's broken, the cause and effect is much easier to see and therefore easier to treat.

This psychological overkill, in my opinion, represents the largest obstacle blocking the path toward greater advances in the treatment of insomnia. When patients say something is wrong with their sleep, then I accept something is wrong with their sleep. My task as a clinician and researcher is to find out what that something is. So, I start as discussed in this book, with the concept of sleep quality, which regrettably 25 years later, many practitioners still avoid taking into account or even discussing with their insomnia patients.

Among those patients who commonly confuse sleep quantity with the concept of quality, many doctors and therapists also have become accustomed to thinking about correcting sleep quantity complaints with drugs or psychotherapy or cognitive-behavioral therapy. In our experience, however, even if insomnia improves with these methods, a sleep quality problem may persist, particularly in those who have had sleep problems for years or who would describe their insomnia as moderate or severe.

Because we invariably asked insomniacs about the quality of their sleep and probed this area in great depth, we are fortunately discovering surprising connections between insomnia and physical sleep disorders. Most commonly we see sleep apnea, now designated as sleep-disordered breathing or SDB for short.

We have researched this SDB connection to insomnia in several types of patients. For example, we conducted studies with rape survivors and victims of childhood sexual abuse; we've studied evacuees following a natural disaster; and we've worked with adults who experienced various types of criminal victimization. In addition, I have also worked in commercial sleep clinics where many insomniacs come for treatment. In all these settings, we have been surprised to learn the majority of insomniacs with moderate to severe sleep complaints also suffer sleep-disordered breathing.

Sometimes SDB takes the obvious form of sleep apnea

where airflow during sleep is so obstructed it actually ceases for 10 seconds or longer. In more instances, SDB takes the form of upper airway resistance, which means the flow of air did not stop, but it was noticeably constrained as if it were drawn through a tube whose diameter was too small to permit sufficient flow. Regardless of the exact description of the breathing disruption, the important point is individuals with either type of SDB suffer from hundreds of nocturnal brain arousals or frank awakenings all through their sleep. As such, they are not really sleeping in a consolidated manner. Instead, they are waking up and returning to sleep hundreds of times per night.

Logically, one might assume SDB ought to be one of the first things to consider in searching for the cause of insomnia. This approach has not been adopted routinely for one very good reason: a large number of people with SDB never develop insomnia but instead suffer from chronic sleepiness. In other words, robbed of their sleep through hundreds of awakenings, their response is classic sleep deprivation. They are exhausted and sleepy all day and all night long and never have any difficulty going or returning to sleep. Because this behavior fits the classic definition of sleep apnea, most physicians have become accustomed to thinking a patient without sleepiness cannot have sleep- disordered breathing.

We predict there is a different and very large group of patients who suffer these SDB-induced awakenings, but they develop insomnia instead of daytime sleepiness. We make this prediction because we have documented rates of SDB between 50 and 90% in our research participants who enrolled in our programs for the treatment of insomnia, and we consistently observe this diagnosis in more than 75% of insomniacs presenting to our sleep clinics.

To reiterate, why these awakenings promote insomnia in one

person and sleepiness in another is an interesting question to be researched in the future, but more importantly, our curiosity has been further piqued by successfully curing insomnia in patients treated for their sleep-disordered breathing. Our 2019 peer-reviewed paper published in the *The Lancet* journal *EClinicalMedicine* demonstrated how insomnia can be cured with a PAP device, the treatment for SDB. You can find the study online: "Prospective Randomized Controlled Trial on the Efficacy of Continuous Positive Airway Pressure and Adaptive Servo-Ventilation in the Treatment of Chronic Complex Insomnia."

SDB treatment is not as easy as taking a pill, and it may even appear threatening to some insomniacs. Nonetheless, we have worked with hundreds of research and clinic patients whose insomnia was markedly reduced or completely eliminated by successful application of SDB treatment.

Remarkably, many of these insomniacs gained benefits from CBT, yet gained still greater benefits by treating SDB and further reducing their insomnia.

Most of these patients learned how to use a breathing mask that provides positive airway pressure that keeps the diameter of your breathing tube wide open during the night. It eliminates snoring or any other subtle breathing disruption, such as upper airway resistance, and in so doing, it eliminates the hundreds of brain arousals and awakenings throughout the night. For these patients, it appears that fixing the sleep breathing problem was the direct path to fixing the sleep quality problem. Once sleep quality was enhanced, many of these patients reported their insomnia was cured.

Thomas Paine said, "Time makes more converts than reason." And, in my professional clinical and research experience, I appreciate it will take a considerable period of time for patients, doctors and therapists to recognize that physical sleep disorders play an important role in causing or worsening insomnia. My objective as a clinician and a researcher is to get the reasons out there, so people will have the opportunity to judge for themselves whether or not this pathway is relevant to their problem. Perhaps more importantly, this new knowledge will assist clinicians in recognizing the importance of treating sleep-disordered breathing among people complaining of insomnia.

For your own education, we would encourage you to consider my latest book, *Life Saving Sleep: New Horizons in Mental Health Treatment,* available wherever books are sold.

ENDNOTES

QUICK GUIDE

If you are considering whether sleep-disordered breathing underlies your insomnia, please consider the following practical steps in pursuing such an evaluation. Also, my new book, *Life Saving Sleep: New Horizons in Mental Health Treatment*, covers these aspects in great depth, but the following info will prime you with a few key terms.

Self-assessment

Spend time reading about sleep-disordered breathing to communicate easily with healthcare providers who often will know less than you do. If you do *not* snore, it's important to read about upper airway resistance syndrome (UARS) as this SDB variant could still be in play. Again, few healthcare providers know anything about UARS. Ideally, you learn so much from your own reading, you can make your own self-assessment before contacting a healthcare provider.

Contacting a Healthcare Provider

Unless you are independently wealthy or pay for an insurance plan that permits direct access to specialists, I believe it will prove invaluable to make contact with a primary care provider, that is, your regular doctor, to pursue treatment for SDB. Certainly, if you have a managed care insurance program, you would be required to do so. If you can convince or persuade your primary doctor your chances for SDB are much higher than he or she would have imagined, then you will have made a formidable ally in your attempt to get adequate assessment and treatment for SDB once you are referred to a sleep specialist.

Sleep Specialist
Sleep medicine centers and labs may present the thorniest areas on your path forward, because many sincere, dedicated but overworked sleep specialists have not kept abreast of the knowledge showing a relationship between insomnia and SDB. Worse, many sleep specialists are still skeptical or unaware of the advances in respiratory assessment technology to measure subtle breathing conditions such as UARS.

In other words, once you get an appointment with a sleep specialist, you may still need to convince this doctor to conduct a sleep study, and you may need to clarify how the sleep lab captures and scores all types of breathing events, including the UARS component. You can see how thorny these circumstances could get, because it might make the doctor feel like he or she is being pushed around by someone who appears to know too much. In my years as an internist, emergency medicine physician and sleep specialist, I've always welcomed motivated patients who had done homework before their appointments. However, I know from practical experience the key to success in such encounters is DIPLOMACY. Sleep specialists are becoming inundated with requests for services and are being pushed by managed care and hospital administrators to provide faster, less comprehensive medical care. As long as you offer your self-assessment with respect and sincerity, most physicians of any type are willing to listen and consider your needs at least in theory.

Treatment Options

I advise all SDB patients to try the breathing mask first because even though it might be uncomfortable, it gives you the opportunity to experience high quality sleep almost immediately. This approach is worth its weight in gold because once you actually experience what happens when breathing disruption is removed from your sleep, it greatly increases your motivation to follow through on whatever treatment approach you choose.

For fairly overweight individuals the breathing mask almost always appears to be the best option. For people who are normal or under weight, oral appliances are often effective and sometimes curative of insomnia. But in each of these instances, remember the marketplace offers various types of breathing masks and pressurized air machines and various types of oral appliances. You get what you pay for, so always consider the possibility you will need to make adjustments to the equipment you are using. Or, you may discover a need for new, more advanced equipment if things are not improving as you think they might. In such instances, trial and error during an interval of one to several months may be needed to optimize your treatment.

Conclusion

New advances in SDB treatment are promoted several times per year as the medical profession and interested entrepreneurs appreciate sleep-disordered breathing is incredibly prevalent. Based on this new research emphasis, more people will gain awareness of the connection between SDB and insomnia. If you seek to stay current on this topic, please look for our new research articles as well those of other researchers in this blossoming field of sleep medicine. And, you can also check for regular updates through my Substack newsletter at www.fastasleep.substack.com and my professional website www.barrykrakowmd.com, the latter of which also offering personalized sleep coaching services through video conferencing.

Acknowledgments

I want to thank my wife, Jessica, for steadfastly assisting in the development of this new version of the earlier book, including all facets of editorial review, revisions, proof-reading, and preparation of the manuscript and design cover.

ABOUT THE AUTHOR

B arry Krakow, M.D. is a board-certified internist and sleep disorders specialist. He previously owned and operated Maimonides Sleep Arts & Sciences, Ltd. for 20 years and remains the principal investigator of the non-profit 501(c)(3) research center, the Sleep & Human Health Institute. He has conducted more than 30 years of treatment research on nightmares, insomnia and sleep-disordered breathing with a special focus on those also diagnosed with mental health disorders, including anxiety, depression and posttraumatic stress disorder. His work has led to the recognition of very high rates of sleep-disordered breathing in mental health patients who complain of chronic sleep problems. Dr. Krakow's current work includes training psychiatry residents in clinical approaches to sleep medicine at the Gateway Behavioral Community Service Board psychiatry residency program. His most recent book, *Life Saving Sleep: New Horizons in Mental Health Treatment* offers a much-needed handbook for the mental health community, both patients and professionals alike, who seek to understand the full scope, complexity and influence of sleep disorders on mental illness; available at www.lifesavingsleep.com or wherever books are sold. Last, he regularly posts on his Substack newsletter at www.fastasleep.substack.com and offers professional sleep health coaching services at www.barrykrakowmd.com. He lives in Savannah, Georgia with his wife and two dogs.

www.ingramcontent.com/pod-product-compliance
Lightning Source LLC
Chambersburg PA
CBHW032044040426
42334CB00038B/659